Look After Yourself

Healthy Hair

Angela Royston

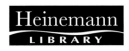
Heinemann
LIBRARY

www.heinemann.co.uk/library
Visit our website to find out more information about **Heinemann Library** books.

To order:
☎ Phone 44 (0) 1865 888066
🖹 Send a fax to 44 (0) 1865 314091
💻 Visit the Heinemann Bookshop at www.heinemann.co.uk/library to browse our catalogue and order online.

First published in Great Britain by Heinemann Library, Halley Court, Jordan Hill, Oxford OX2 8EJ, part of Harcourt Education.
Heinemann is a registered trademark of Harcourt Education Ltd.

Editorial: Sarah Eason and Kathy Peltan
Design: Dave Oakley, Arnos Design
Picture Research: Helen Reilly, Arnos Design
Production: Edward Moore

Originated by Dot Gradations Ltd
Printed and bound in Hong Kong and China by South China

ISBN 0 431 18025 3 (hardback)
07 06 05 04 03
10 9 8 7 6 5 4 3 2 1

ISBN 0 431 18035 0 (paperback)
08 07 06 05 04
10 9 8 7 6 5 4 3 2 1

British Library Cataloguing in Publication Data
Royston, Angela
Healthy hair. – (Look after yourself)
1.Hair – Care and hygiene – Juvenile literature
I.Title
646.7'24

A full catalogue record for this book is available from the British Library.

Acknowledgements
The publishers would like to thank the following for permission to reproduce photographs: Bubbles p.**13** (Angela Hampton), p.**18** (Nick Hanna), p.**23** (Lucy Tizard), p.**25** (Frans Rombout); Gareth Boden p.**14**; Getty Images p.**9** (Pascal Crapet), p.**19** (David Madison), p.**20** (Maria Taglienti); Last Resort p.**26** (Jo Makin); Martin Sookias p.**24**; Photodisc pp.**8**, **15**; Powerstock p.**7**; Science Photo Library p. **22** (BSIP PIR); Trevor Clifford pp.**4**, **5**, **6**, **10**, **11**, **12**, **16**, **17**, **21**, **27**.

Cover photograph reproduced with permission of Bananastock.

The publishers would like to thank David Wright for his assistance in the preparation of this book.

Every effort has been made to contact copyright holders of any material reproduced in this book. Any omissions will be rectified in subsequent printings if notice is given to the publishers.

Contents

Words written in bold, **like this**, are explained in the Glossary.

Your body

Your body is made up of many different parts, such as your skin, your hair, your heart and your ears. Each part works in a different way.

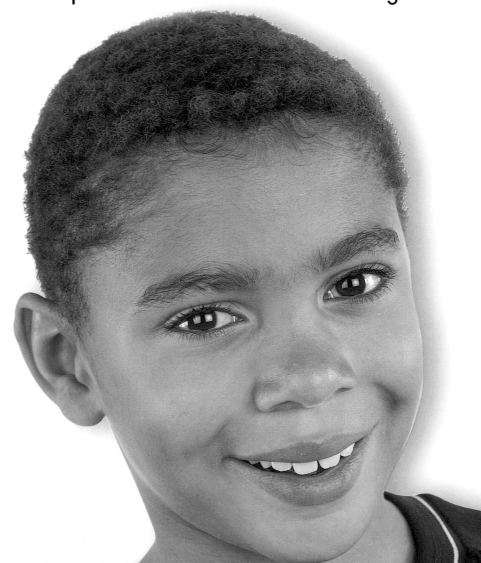

The skin on your head is called your **scalp**. The hair on your head grows from your scalp. This book is about your hair and your scalp.

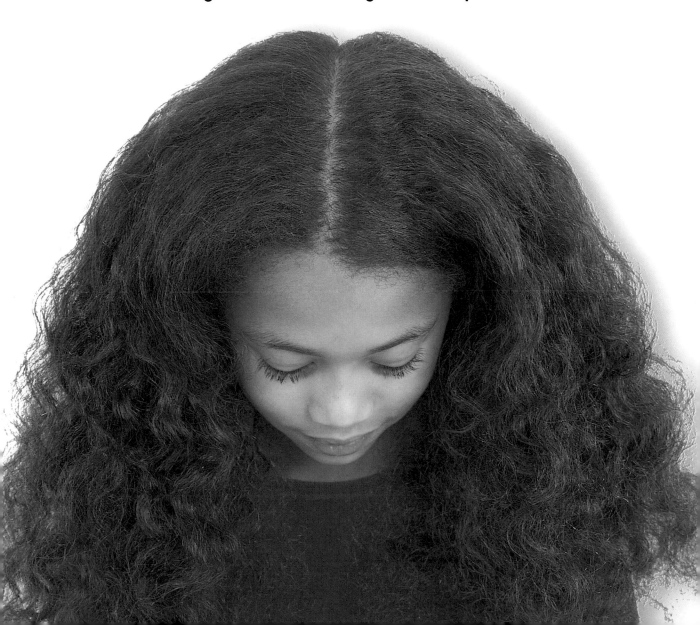

Your hair

Hair helps to keep your head warm. Your brain is inside your head and it works better when it is warm. Hair also affects the way you look.

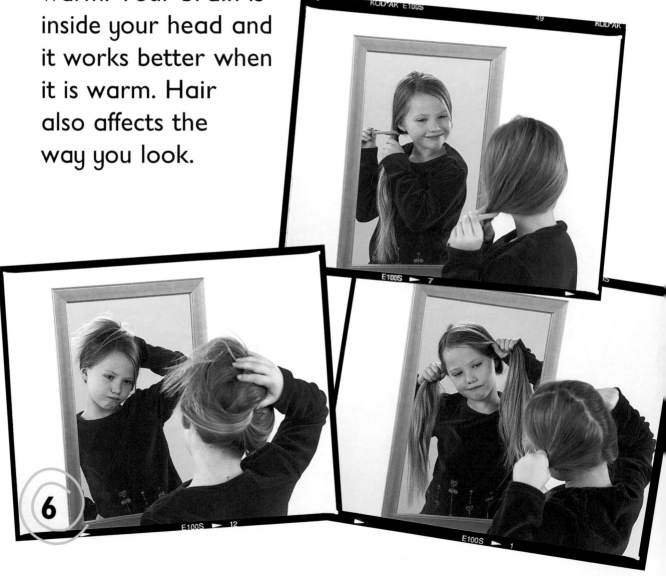

Some people have black hair. Others have red or blonde hair. Some people have curly hair. Others have straight or wavy hair.

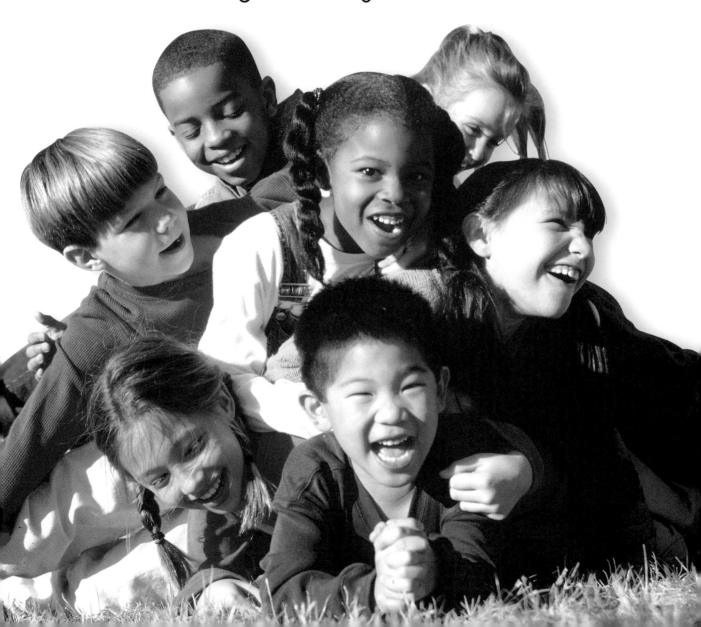

Look after your hair

You need to look after your hair to keep it looking good. Healthy, shiny hair looks better than dirty, dull hair. Clean hair feels better too.

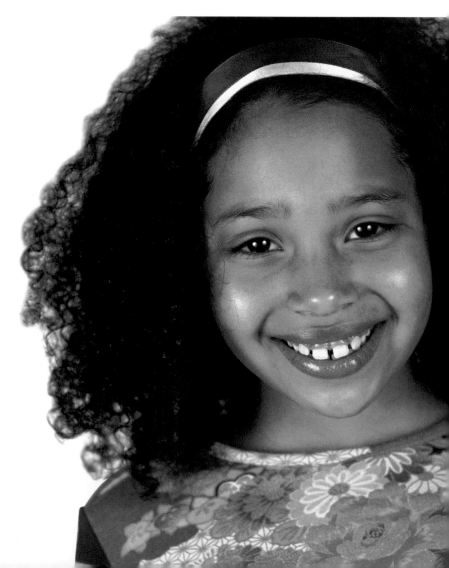

If you do not look after your hair, it will become **tangled** and dirty. Your hair will get in your eyes and it will make your face feel itchy.

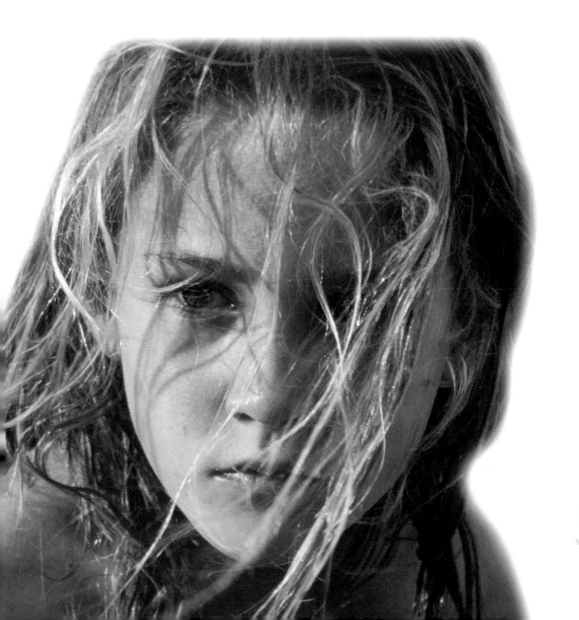

Brush and comb

Brush or comb your hair when you get up in the morning. Brushing and combing **untangles** the hair and makes you feel fresher.

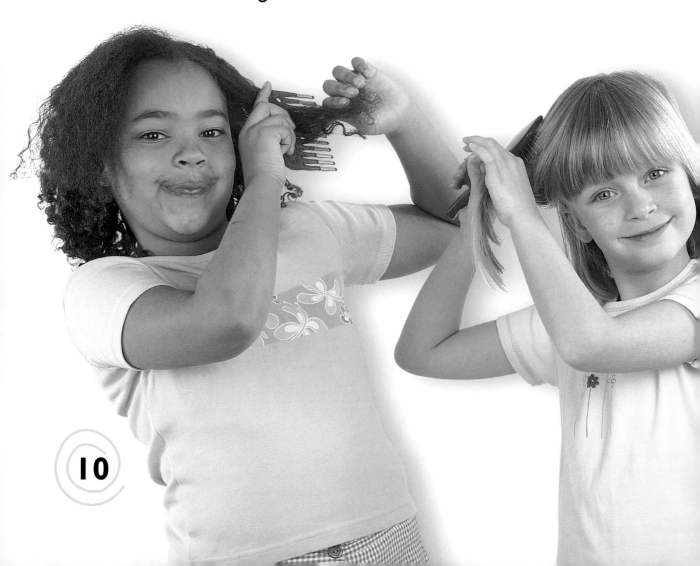

The wind blows your hairs into knots and **tangles**. Brushing or combing them out can hurt. Hold the hair above the tangle before you comb it – this will stop it hurting.

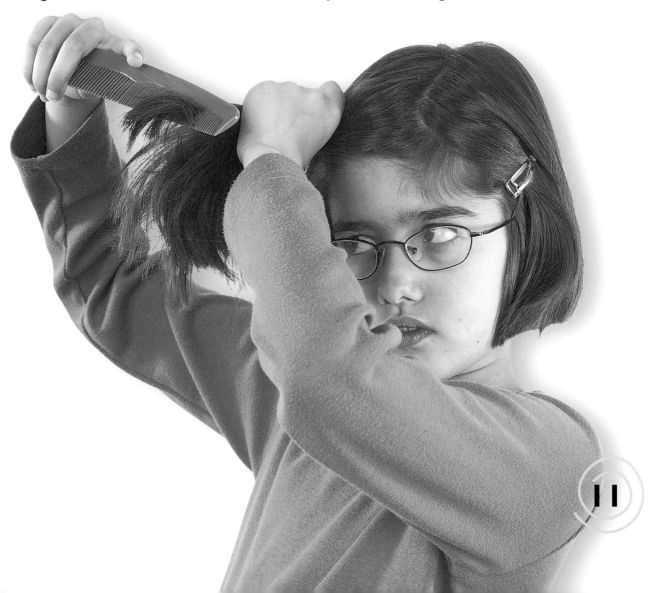

Neat and tidy

Long hair does not stay tidy for long. Some girls use bands or put their hair into **plaits** to keep it neat.

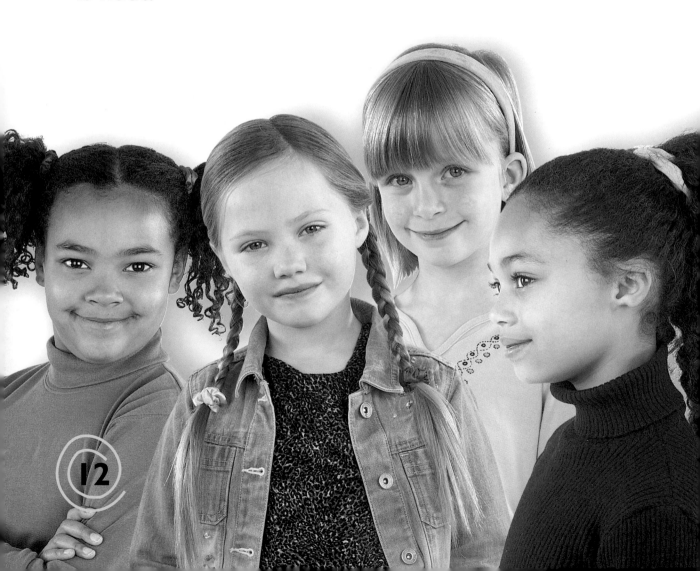

12

You should have your hair cut every few months. Cutting off the ends of your hair keeps it healthier and neater. Do not cut your own hair!

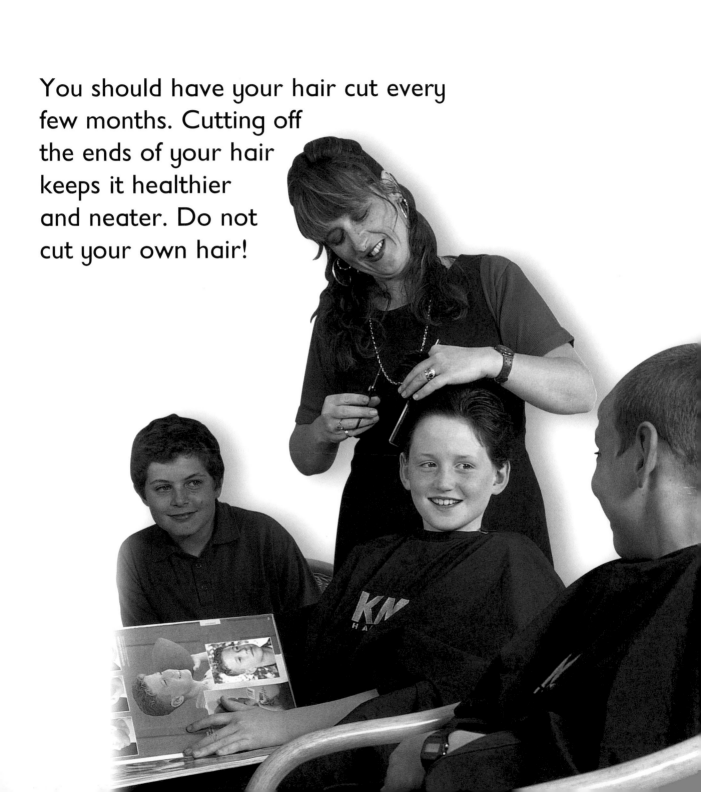

Wash your hair

Washing your hair cleans your **scalp** and your hair. It helps to stop your scalp getting itchy. You need to wash your hair with **shampoo** at least once a week.

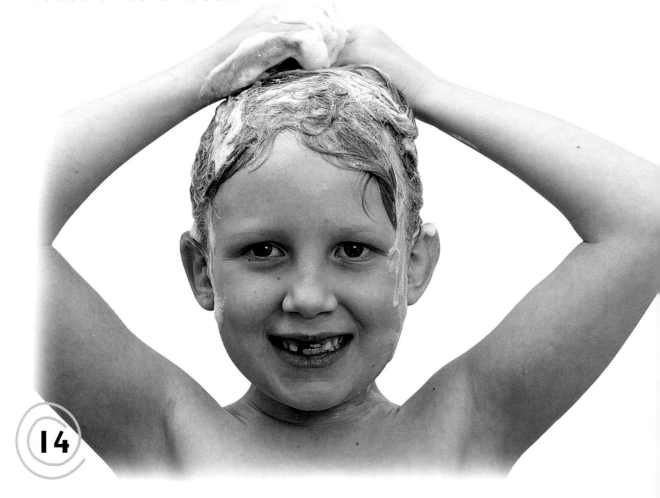

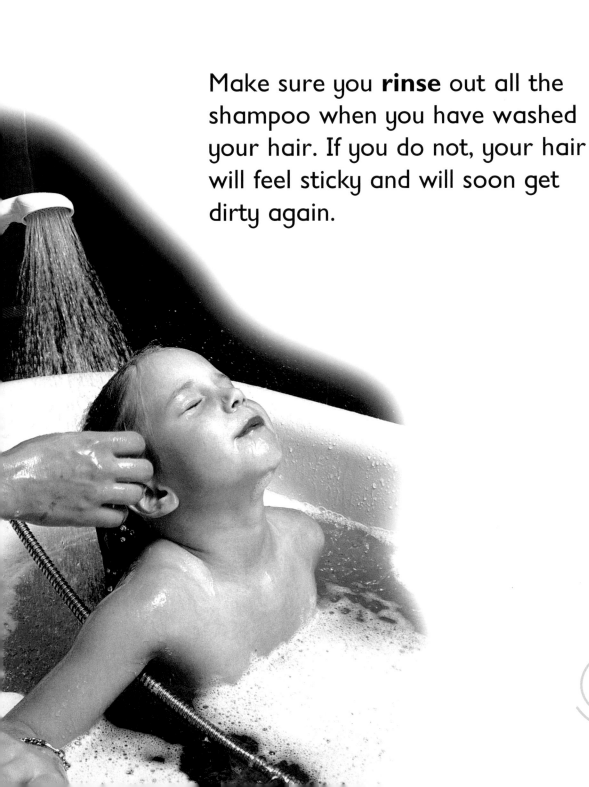

Make sure you **rinse** out all the shampoo when you have washed your hair. If you do not, your hair will feel sticky and will soon get dirty again.

Dry or oily hair?

Your hair has its own **natural oil**. The oil keeps your hair shiny. Some people have more natural oil than others. Use a **shampoo** that suits your hair.

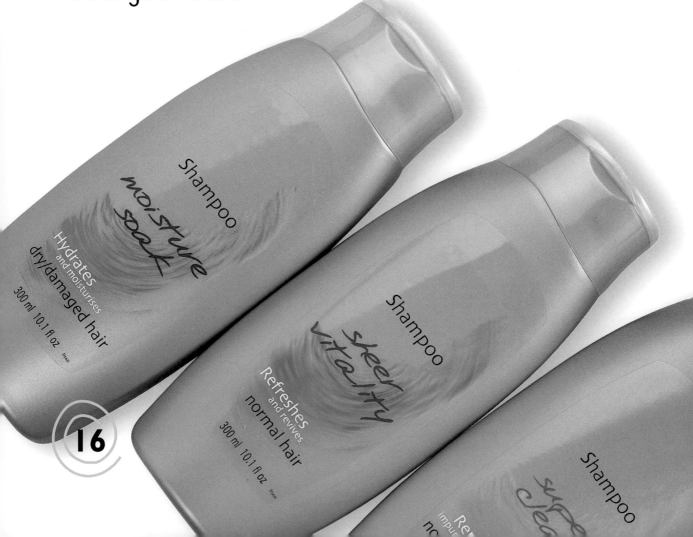

Shampoo

moisture soak

Hydrates
and moisturises

dry/damaged hair

300 ml 10.1 fl oz

Shampoo

sheer vitality

Refreshes
and revives

normal hair

300 ml 10.1 fl oz

Shampoo

If your hair is very fine or dry, you can use a **conditioner**. The conditioner makes your hair more shiny and easy to comb. Some shampoos contain conditioner, too.

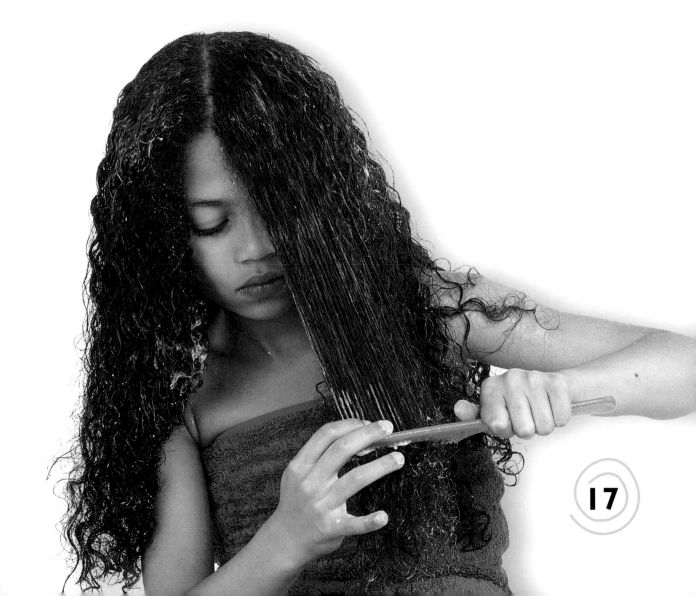

Protect your hair

The Sun can make your hair dry out. Wear a sunhat to protect your hair from hot sunshine. **Chemicals** in the water in a swimming pool can also make your hair dry out.

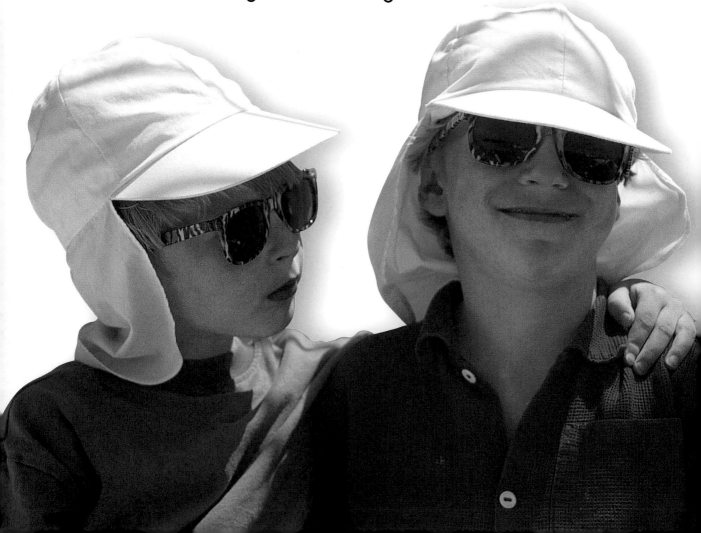

Wash your hair after swimming. It will wash out the chemicals in the swimming pool water. You can protect your hair with a swimming cap, too.

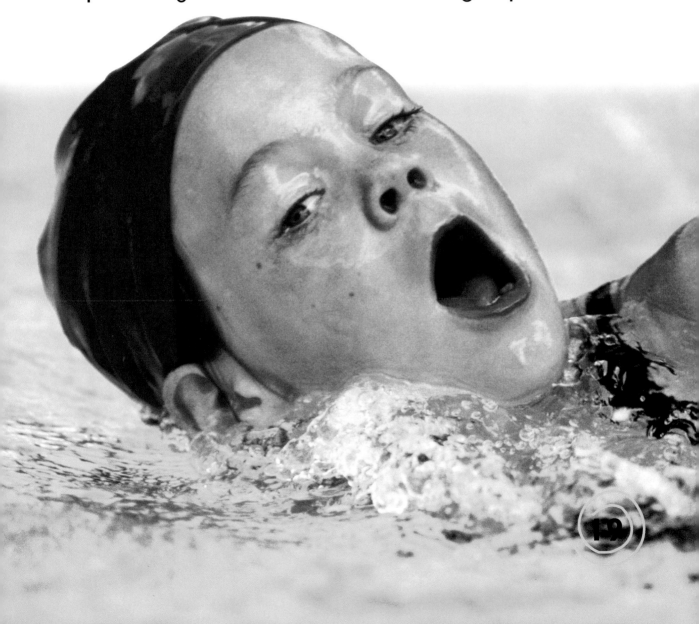

Dry scalp

The skin on your **scalp** may become dry and covered with small white flakes. When you shake your hair, some of the flakes fall out.

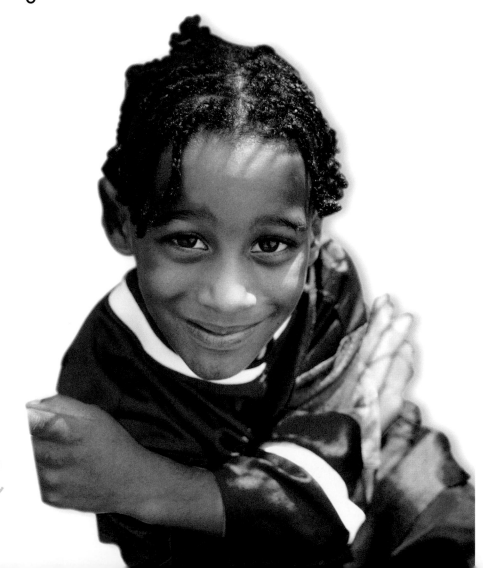

The white flakes are tiny pieces of dead skin from your scalp. You can use a special **shampoo** to get rid of the white flakes and make your scalp less dry. Make sure you wash all the shampoo from your hair, too.

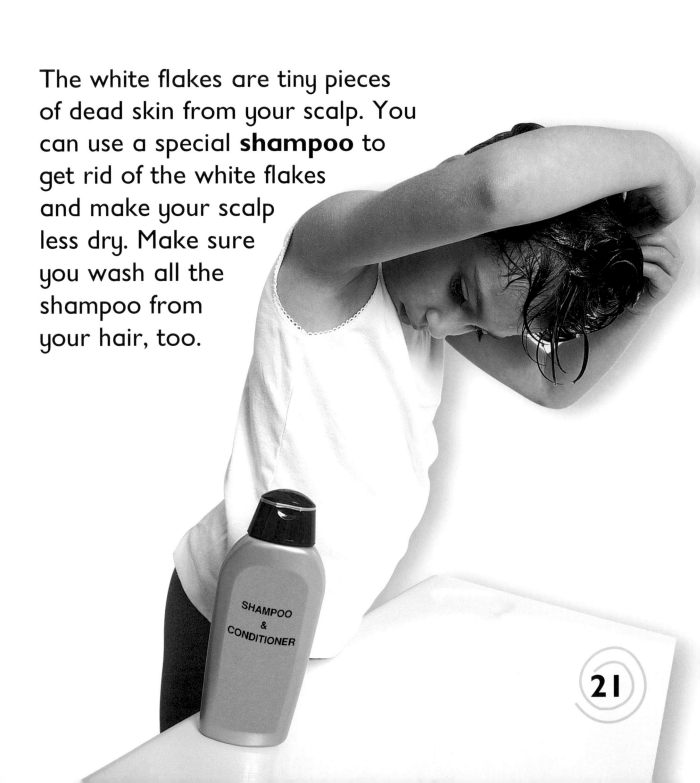

SHAMPOO & CONDITIONER

Head lice

If your head is very itchy, you may have **head lice**. Head lice are insects that spread easily from one person's hair to another person's hair.

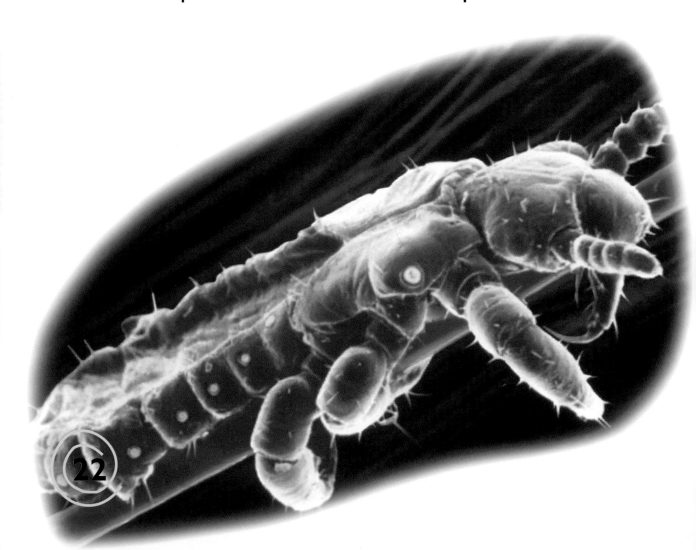

Ask an adult to check your hair for **nits**.
Nits are the eggs of the head lice. They look
like small white flecks, but you cannot
shake them out because they are attached
to the hair.

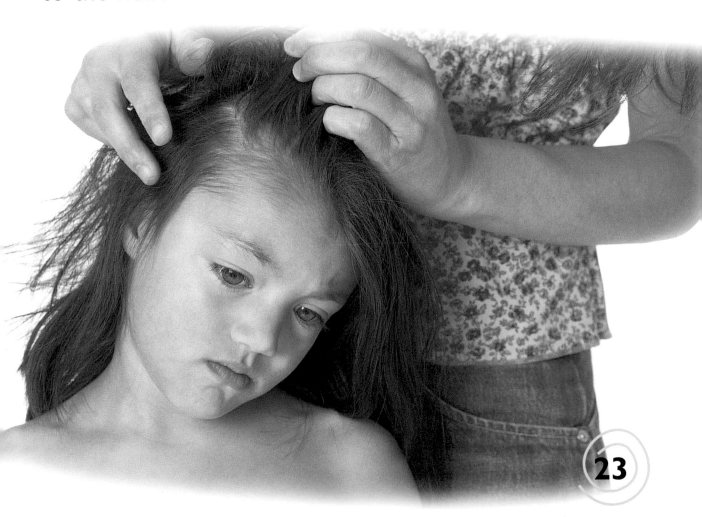

Getting rid of head lice

You have to use a special **shampoo** to kill **head lice**. If you have head lice, tell your teacher. Everyone in your class and their families should use the shampoo, too.

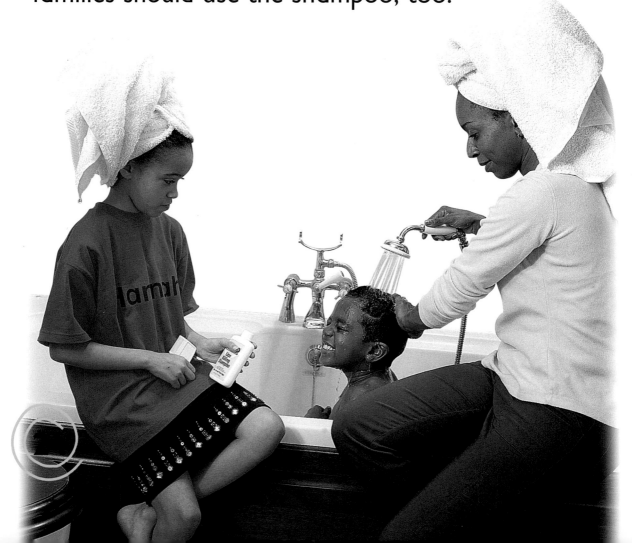

Once the lice are dead you can comb them out with a special comb. The teeth of the comb are very close together, so the lice cannot slip through them.

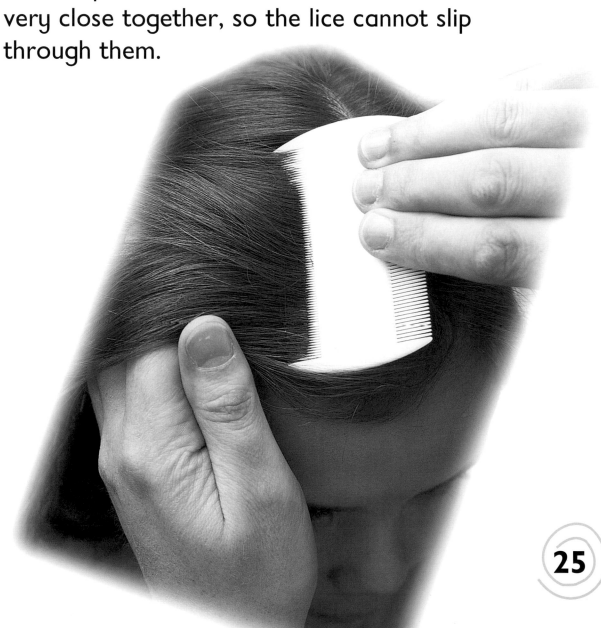

Getting things out of your hair

Sometimes things get stuck in your hair. Jam, honey or ice cream can make your hair sticky. You have to wash your hair to get them out.

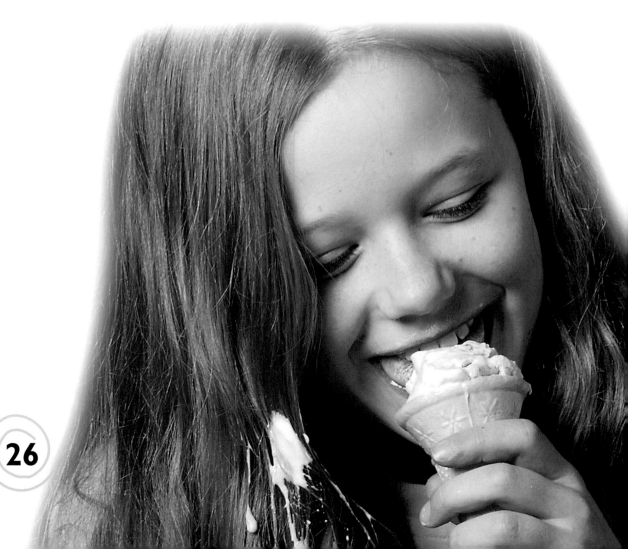

Some things cannot be washed out. If you get glue or chewing gum stuck in your hair, you will have to ask an adult to cut off that piece of hair.

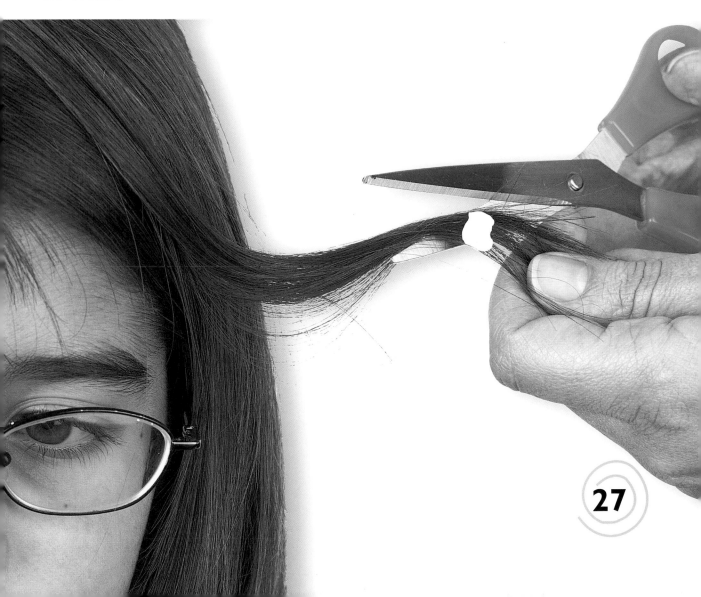

It's a fact!

About a hundred of the hairs on your head fall out every day, but do not worry – you have about 80,000 hairs on your head altogether. Brushing your hair helps to brush away the hairs that have already fallen out.

Children's hair grows faster than adults' hair. Adults' hair grows nearly one and a half centimetres a month.

Each hair grows from a tiny pouch in your skin called a hair **follicle**. After a hair has dropped out, the follicle rests for a few months. Then a new hair begins to grow.

Each single hair grows for between two and six years before it falls out. This means that most people cannot grow their hair longer than about 80 centimetres. Very few people can grow their hair a metre long and keep it healthy.

If your hair is never cut, the ends of your hairs may split. **Split ends** make your hair look untidy and wispy.

Some people have strong hair. Others have fine hair. You can help to make your hair look stronger and healthier by having it cut regularly.

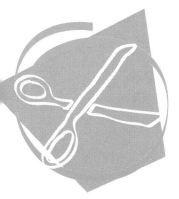

Glossary

chemical substance, for example chlorine, that is put into the water of swimming pools

conditioner creamy liquid that makes the hair less dry and more smooth and shiny

follicle small pouch in the skin from which a hair grows

head lice small insects that live in the hair and feed on blood from the scalp

natural oil greasy liquid made in your scalp that keeps your hair shiny and bendy

nits empty eggs of head lice that are left behind when the lice have hatched

plait way of arranging hair in three strands that are woven together. A plait is also called a braid.

rinse wash with clean water

scalp   layer of skin that covers the top and back of the head and from which hair grows

shampoo   soapy liquid that is used for washing hair

split end   when part of a hair splits to form a short, extra end

tangled   twisted and muddled together

untangle   make free from knots and muddles

Find out more

Healthy Living: Healthy Hair by Constance Milburn (Wayland, 1990)

It's Catching: Head Lice by Angela Royston (Heinemann Library, 2002)

Look After Yourself: Your Hair by Claire Llewellyn (Watts, 2002)

Safe and Sound: Clean and Healthy by Angela Royston (Heinemann Library, 2000)

Taking Care of My Hair by Elizabeth Vogel (PowerKids Press, 2001)

Index

Science@School | Book 6F

How we see things

A brief history

TODAY... 1849 French physicist, Armand-Hippolyte-Louis Fizeau measures the speed of light in air at 315km/sec... 1847 John Draper, in England, shows that as something is heated it first turns dull red, then orange, yellow and white, no matter what substance it is made from... 1841 German scientist, Carl Gauss explains how to work out the way light behaves when it passes through a lens. This allows lenses to be designed on scientific principles... 1840 Alexander Becquerel, in France, shows that light can be used to make electricity... 1704 Isaac Newton writes a book on light called *Optics*... 1665 Newton discovers that white light is made from a mixture of colours... 1621 In Holland, Willebrord Snell finds that light can be bent as it passes through glass. He sets this out as Snell's Law... 1607 Gallileo, in Italy, builds the first telescope that can be used for looking at planets and stars... 1270 Polish mathematician, Witelo shows that light rays enter the eye from objects around us. Before this people thought that the eye sent out beams of light like a torch... 1010 Abu 'Ali Al-Hasan explains how lenses work and develops a mirror whose design is still used in modern telescopes... 140 Claudius Ptolemy, in Egypt, writes a book in Greek on light and optics. The Greek version is lost, and Western scientists only find out about the book when an Arabic version is translated into Latin 1,000 years later... 100 Hero, of Alexandria, writes a book about light and mirrors...

For more information visit www.science-at-school.com

Dr Brian Knapp

Word list

These are some science words that you should look out for as you go through the book. They are shown using CAPITAL letters.

BEAM
A broad band or shaft of light such as that produced by a torch. Sunbeams are beams of sunlight.

CELL
The small building blocks that make up all living things. Cells are specialised to help the body in various ways. Rods and cones are cells in the eye that are sensitive to light and colour.

CONCAVE MIRROR
A curved mirror in which the middle is further away from you than the edge. The inside of a dish-shaped mirror is concave.

CONVEX MIRROR
A curved mirror in which the middle is closer to you than the edge. A bulging mirror is convex.

ECLIPSE
The shadow made when the Moon comes between the Sun and the Earth. This is called an eclipse of the Sun. At this time the Moon is seen in silhouette as it casts a shadow over part of the Earth.

FIELD OF VIEW
The angle you can see. If the angle is narrow, you have a narrow field of view.

FOCUS
(a) To see things clearly.
(b) The point at which rays of light meet.

GLARE
Light that is so bright it makes you squint. Glare is often caused by light reflecting from a mirror-like surface, such as water or cars.

LASER
A machine able to produce a very concentrated beam of light.

LENS
A curved piece of transparent material, such as glass, that causes light rays to bend.

LIGHT YEAR
The distance light travels in a year (nearly 10 trillion km).

OPAQUE
Something that light cannot get through. Opposite of transparent.

PINHOLE
A small hole through which light is shone. A pinhole can be used to make a sharp image.

RAY
A single line or narrow band of light. Light rays are much narrower than beams of light. Their main use in science is in tracing the path of light.

REFLECT
To bounce from a surface. Light reflects in much the same way as sound.

SHADOW
A dark or partly-dark shape that is cast by an object when it blocks out rays of light.

SILHOUETTE
The black outline of an object when seen from its shadow.

SOURCE OF LIGHT
Something that gives out light. The Sun and other stars are the largest sources of light. Street lamps, fires, oil and gas lamps and torches are other examples of sources of light.

SPECTRUM
The name given to all of the colours of visible light.

TRANSPARENT
Something that light will pass through easily. Opposite of opaque.

2